Managing Diabetes

A Journey to Healing for Newly Diagnosed Patients with Real-life Survivor Stories

by

Collin Sherwood, MD

Table of Content

To those who face the daily battle against diabetes with courage and determination, this book is dedicated. Your resilience inspires us all to strive for a healthier tomorrow. To the survivors whose stories illuminate these pages, your journeys remind us that hope and perseverance are powerful allies in the fight against diabetes. May this guide offer support, insight, and the promise of freedom to all who seek it.

Introduction

Diabetes affects millions of lives worldwide, presenting a daily challenge that demands attention, resilience, and proactive management. This book is a comprehensive resource designed to empower individuals with the knowledge, strategies, and inspiration needed to take control of their diabetes journey.

Within these pages, you'll find a wealth of information, from understanding the fundamentals of diabetes to implementing practical lifestyle changes that can make a significant difference in managing the condition. We delve into nutrition, exercise, medication management, and emotional well-being, providing actionable insights tailored to the diverse needs and circumstances of individuals living with diabetes.

Moreover, "Fighting Diabetes" goes beyond clinical advice, incorporating real-life survivor stories that offer encouragement, insight, and solidarity. These narratives illustrate the diverse paths to managing and even overcoming diabetes, demonstrating that with determination and support, achieving freedom from the constraints of diabetes is indeed possible.

Whether you're newly diagnosed, a seasoned veteran in the battle against diabetes, or supporting a loved one on their journey, this book is intended to be your companion, guide, and source of hope. Together, let's embark on a journey toward greater health, vitality, and freedom from diabetes.

Let the journey begin.

Chapter 1

The Origin of Diabetes

Diabetes has a fascinating historical backdrop that spans centuries. Ancient civilizations such as Egypt and Greece documented symptoms resembling those of diabetes, including excessive thirst and frequent urination. However, it wasn't until the 19th century that significant advancements were made in understanding the condition.

During this period, scientists began to unravel the intricacies of diabetes. One pivotal discovery was the identification of the pancreas's role in regulating blood sugar levels. Researchers observed that individuals with diabetes lacked the ability to produce insulin, a hormone crucial for glucose metabolism. This led to the classification of diabetes into different types, with Type 1 characterized by insufficient insulin production and Type 2 marked by insulin resistance.

As medical knowledge evolved, so did our understanding of diabetes management and treatment. From the discovery of insulin in the early 20th century to the development of oral medications and insulin analogs, scientists have made remarkable strides in improving outcomes for individuals living with diabetes.

》Recent Statistics

Despite these advancements, diabetes remains a pressing global health issue, with profound implications for individuals and healthcare systems alike. In the United States alone, diabetes affects over *34 million people*, encompassing both diagnosed and undiagnosed cases. This figure represents approximately 10% of the American population and describes the magnitude of the diabetes epidemic.

Moreover, the prevalence of diabetes continues to rise, driven by factors such as sedentary lifestyles, poor dietary habits, and an aging population. Each year, an estimated *1.5 million new cases* are diagnosed, adding to the already substantial burden of diabetes management and care.

Beyond the personal toll it exacts, diabetes imposes significant economic costs on society. Healthcare expenditures related to diabetes and its complications run into the tens of billions annually, straining healthcare budgets and resources. Furthermore, indirect costs such as lost productivity and disability further compound the socioeconomic impact of diabetes.

In light of these challenges, addressing diabetes requires a concerted effort from healthcare professionals, policymakers, and the broader community. By raising awareness, promoting prevention strategies, and improving access to care, we can mitigate the impact of diabetes and enhance the quality of life for affected individuals.

As we journey through the chapters ahead, we will explore various aspects of diabetes management, from lifestyle modifications to pharmacological interventions. By equipping readers with knowledge and resources, I aim to empower individuals to take control of their health and effectively manage diabetes for a brighter, healthier future.

Chapter 2

Recognizing the Early Signs of Diabetes

In the early stages, diabetes can manifest with subtle symptoms that are easily overlooked or attributed to other factors. Recognizing these early signs is crucial for timely diagnosis and intervention. Let's delve into the often unnoticed symptoms of diabetes and shed light on its hidden challenges.

》*Early Symptoms*

Diabetes can present with a range of symptoms that may vary in severity and duration. Some of the early signs include:

1. Increased Thirst and Urination: One of the hallmark symptoms of diabetes is polyuria, or excessive urination, often accompanied by increased thirst. This occurs as the kidneys work overtime to eliminate excess glucose from the bloodstream.

2. Fatigue and Weakness: Individuals with diabetes may experience persistent fatigue and weakness, even after adequate rest. Fluctuating blood sugar levels can disrupt energy metabolism, leading to feelings of exhaustion.

3. Unexplained Weight Loss: Despite maintaining regular eating habits, some individuals with diabetes may experience unexplained weight loss. This occurs as the body breaks down muscle and fat tissue for energy in the absence of sufficient insulin.

4. Blurred Vision: Changes in blood sugar levels can affect the shape of the lens in the eye, leading to blurred or distorted vision. This symptom may come and go, making it easy to dismiss as temporary eye strain.

5. Slow Wound Healing: Diabetes can impair the body's ability to heal wounds and infections due to reduced circulation and compromised immune function. Minor cuts and bruises may take longer to heal, increasing the risk of complications.

It's important to note that these symptoms may develop gradually over time, making them easy to overlook or dismiss as normal signs of aging or stress. However, ignoring these warning signs can delay diagnosis and exacerbate the progression of diabetes.

》*Highlighting Personal Stories*

Behind the statistics and medical terminology lie the personal stories of individuals grappling with the daily realities of diabetes. These stories offer a glimpse into the hidden struggles and triumphs of those affected by the condition.

From the newly diagnosed teenager learning to navigate insulin injections to the middle-aged professional balancing blood sugar management with a demanding career, each individual's journey with diabetes is unique. Yet, common themes of resilience, adaptation, and perseverance thread through their experiences.

Below is a list of Patient Success stories extracted from Diabetes Center of Excellence (DCOE). The following success stories are intended to provide hope and motivation for all people living with Type 1 or Type 2 diabetes!

June 22, 2023
Jim Cormier

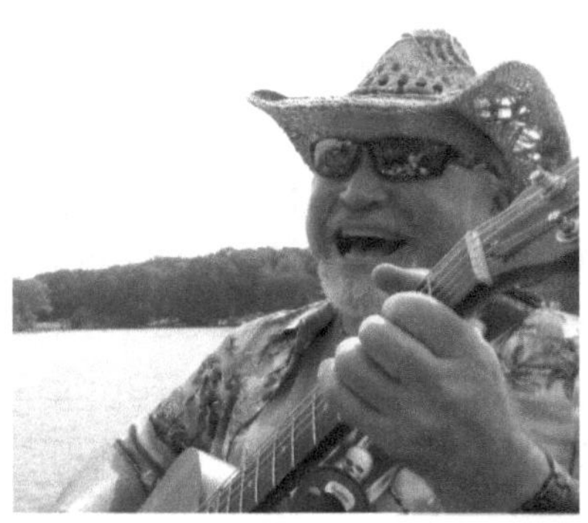

Jim Cormier was diagnosed with type 1 diabetes at two months old in 1967. His new insulin pump & CGM, combined with diabetes education, has led to his first ever A1c below 7%. In this success story he shares what motivated him to finally take control of his diabetes. He has a wonderful relationship with his endocrinologist & nurse practitioner.

December 29, 2022
Michael O'Rourke

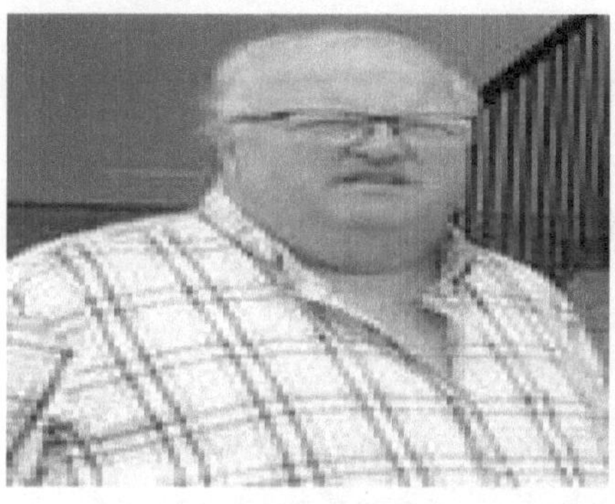

Michael was diagnosed with Type 2 diabetes in his 20's but for more than 40 years has admittedly done nothing to proactively manage it until enrolling for a Care Coach Program at a Diabetes Center. During his first year working with a diabetes coach, his A1c dropped from 8.5% to 6.4%. He credits his new continuous glucose monitor & weekly coaching calls with keeping him on track.

May 18, 2022
Bob Christian

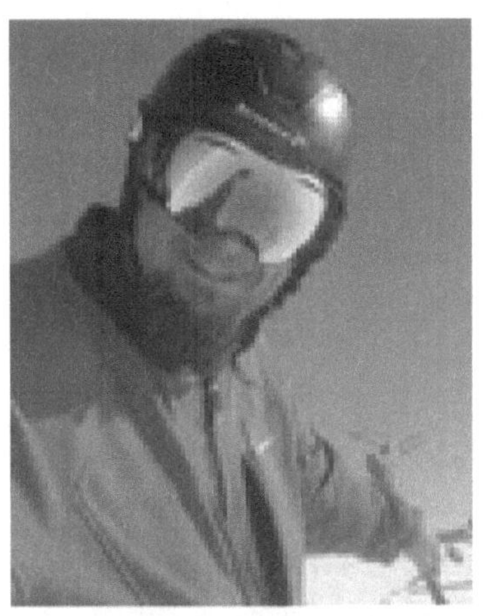

Bob Christian never lets his Type 1 diabetes slow him down. He's an avid kite surfer, who flies large kites to pull him along the water on a board and across fields of snow while wearing skis. His transition to life with diabetes was easier than most because his daughter was diagnosed at 13 years old and had been successfully managing her T1D for more than five years. Meet Bob and learn how he manages his blood sugars while performing stunts on the water and snow.

April 22, 2022
Nan Hilton

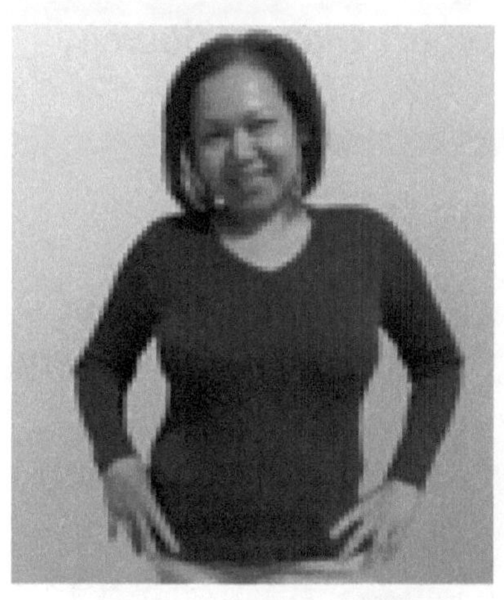

Nan Hilton was diagnosed with Type 2 diabetes at 23 years old. After years of medications and insulin, she made lifestyle modifications resulting in a 90 pound weight loss and she no longer takes any diabetes medications. During a difficult pregnancy, Nan developed severe diabetic retinopathy that required invasive surgery and painful injections. After giving birth she committed to make necessary changes. She started her journey wearing size 16 pants and XL shirts. Today she's down to women's 4/6 pants and small shirts but prefers to wear junior clothing because they fit her better. You'll Learn how she did it.

Peg Olsen 60 Years Type 1 Diabetic Journey
Peg Olsen

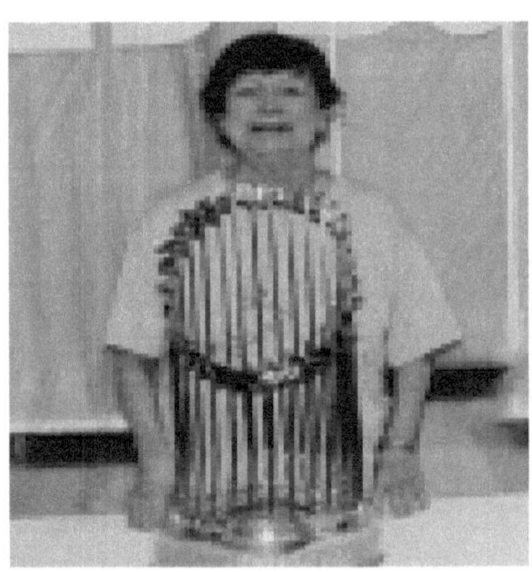

Peg Olsen celebrated her 60th anniversary with Type 1 diabetes during the summer of 2021. She was diagnosed at 9 years old and remembers her mother having to boil her urine on the stove multiple times a day to test her blood sugar. For more than 40 years she chose to manage diabetes with needle injections and tested her blood sugar manually. Finally she agreed to try an insulin pump and continuous glucose monitor in 2002.

March 02, 2022
Taylor Connor Type 1 Diabetes
Taylor Connor

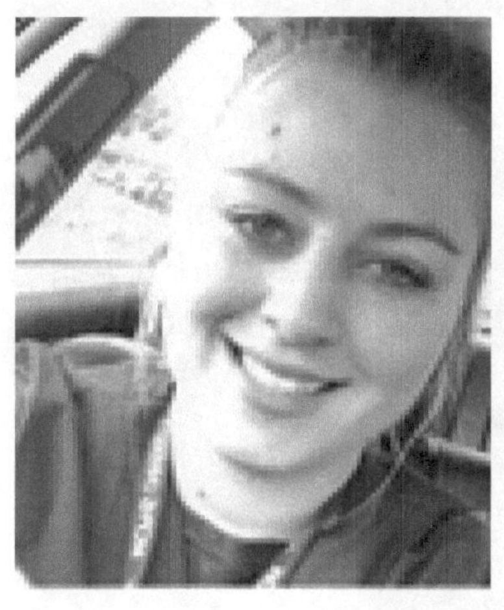

Taylor Connor's journey with Type 1 diabetes has been a long and difficult road. Her A1c reached 15% in 2011 and remained elevated until 2016. That's when she made a personal commitment to her health and started 2022 with an all-time low A1c of 6.4%. Taylor's inspiring story proves it's never too late to take control of diabetes. Using an insulin pump for the first time and adopting a healthy eating lifestyle has changed her life. In addition to improved health, it also resulted in her attending nursing school and today she's a Nurse and plans to become a Diabetes Educator.

February 01, 2022
Andy Nelson Diabetes Success Story
Andrew Nelson

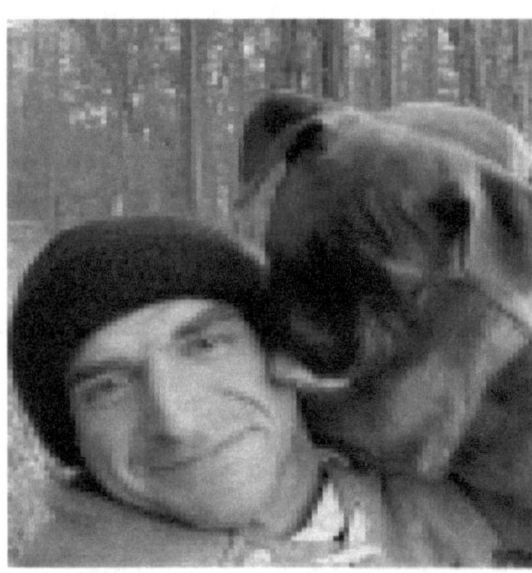

Andrew Nelson is living his second chance. He was diagnosed with

insulin-dependent diabetes following one of many surgeries as the result of pancreatitis and other health issues. He was referred to a Diabetes Center taking multiple daily insulin injections and other oral medications. Today he is no longer taking any medications, including insulin! He credits his care team with helping him become educated about diabetes

management which allowed him to make the
necessary modifications to improve his health.

December 06, 2021
Charles Morse

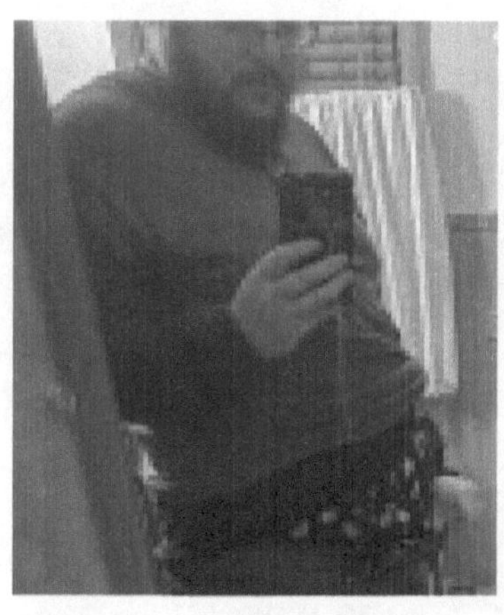

Charles was diagnosed with Type 2 diabetes in 2015 at the age of 30. He was referred to a Diabetes Center in early 2021 because of severe insulin resistance. At the time he was injecting 425 units of insulin each day, but his blood sugars were still above 400 mg/dL, his A1c was 11.0% and his blood pressure was also very high despite taking several medications. In less than a year his diabetes care team helped him to lower his A1c to 7%.

May 01, 2021
Type 1 Diabetes Success Story
Joey

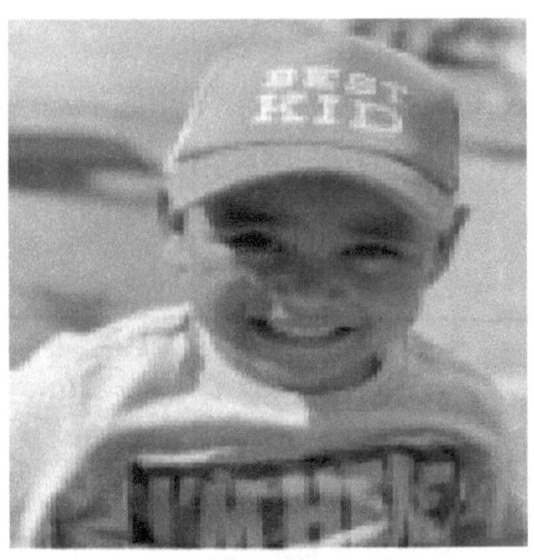

Joey was diagnosed with type 1 diabetes at five years old in August of 2020 during the coronavirus pandemic. At first he was inconsolable but he made incredible progress during his first year. He recognizes high and low blood sugars and knows how to treat them. Joey's mother describes their road from diagnosis, including working closely with his care team and school nurse as challenging but ultimately worth it.

September 03, 2021
kitty Carruthers diabetes success story
Kitty Carruthers

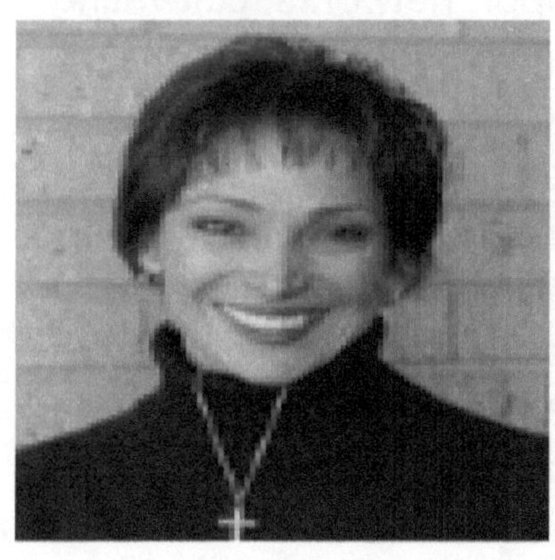

U.S. Olympian and four time National Figure Skating Champion, Kitty Carruthers doesn't allow diabetes to stand in the way of her life. With determination to succeed perfected in international competitions, Kitty is also determined to succeed in staying healthy. Her doctor has been helping her for many years and together they've managed to keep her blood sugars within a healthy range.

For many, managing diabetes is not just about monitoring blood sugar levels and adhering to treatment regimens; it's about facing stigma, overcoming misconceptions, and advocating for better healthcare resources. It's about finding support networks, cultivating resilience, and reclaiming control over one's health and well-being.

By sharing these personal narratives, we honor the voices of those living with diabetes and shed light on the often unseen challenges they confront. Their stories serve as a reminder of the importance of empathy, understanding, and solidarity in the fight against diabetes.

In the chapters ahead, we will continue to explore practical strategies for diabetes management while drawing inspiration from the courage and resilience of individuals who refuse to let diabetes define them. Together, we can empower each other to confront the challenges of diabetes with compassion, determination, and hope.

Chapter 3

Understanding Diabetes Types

Diabetes is not a one-size-fits-all condition. There are different types of diabetes, each with its own characteristics, causes, and management strategies. Let's break down the nuances between Type 1 and Type 2 diabetes and explore the risk factors associated with each type.

》Different Types of Diabetes

Type 1 Diabetes: Type 1 diabetes, often referred to as juvenile diabetes, is an autoimmune condition where the body's immune system mistakenly attacks and destroys insulin-producing cells in the pancreas. As a result, individuals with Type 1 diabetes produce little to no insulin, the hormone responsible for regulating blood sugar levels. This type of diabetes typically develops in childhood or adolescence, but it can occur at any age.

Type 2 Diabetes: Type 2 diabetes is the most common form of diabetes and is characterized by insulin resistance, where the body's cells become less responsive to insulin. Initially, the pancreas produces extra insulin to compensate for this resistance, but over time, it may not be able to keep up with demand. Type 2 diabetes is often linked to lifestyle factors such as obesity, physical inactivity, and unhealthy eating habits. While it primarily affects adults, it is becoming more prevalent in children and adolescents due to rising rates of obesity.

》Insights into Risk Factors

Understanding the risk factors associated with each type of diabetes can help individuals assess their own susceptibility and take proactive steps to mitigate their risk.

- Type 1 Diabetes Risk Factors:

Family history: Having a close relative with Type 1 diabetes increases the risk.

Genetics: Certain genes are associated with an increased susceptibility to Type 1 diabetes.

Environmental factors: Exposure to certain viruses or toxins may trigger the autoimmune response that leads to Type 1 diabetes.

■ Type 2 Diabetes Risk Factors:

Obesity: Being overweight or obese significantly increases the risk of developing Type 2 diabetes.

Sedentary lifestyle: Lack of physical activity and prolonged periods of sitting or inactivity contribute to insulin resistance.

Unhealthy diet: Consuming a diet high in processed foods, sugary beverages, and refined carbohydrates can increase the risk of Type 2 diabetes.

Age: The risk of Type 2 diabetes increases with age, especially after the age of 45.

Family history: Having a family history of Type 2 diabetes raises the likelihood of developing the condition.

By understanding these risk factors, you can make informed choices about your lifestyle, diet, and healthcare practices to reduce your risk of developing diabetes. Regular exercise, a balanced diet, maintaining a healthy weight, and routine medical check-ups are essential components of diabetes prevention and management.

In the upcoming chapters, we will delve deeper into strategies for preventing and managing diabetes, tailored to the specific needs and challenges of each type. Armed with knowledge and awareness, you can take proactive steps towards achieving optimal health and well-being.

Chapter 4

Exposing the Culprits

Diabetes isn't just a result of chance; it's often influenced by lifestyle factors that have become increasingly prevalent in modern society. In this chapter, we'll uncover the culprits behind the rise of diabetes in the U.S. and offer practical tips for you to evaluate and modify your lifestyle choices to reduce your risk.

Let's delve deeper into each of the lifestyle factors contributing to the rise of diabetes in the U.S. and provide more detailed practical tips for you to evaluate and modify your lifestyle choices:

》Identifying Lifestyle Factors

1. Sedentary Habits

Sedentary lifestyles have become increasingly common due to the prevalence of desk jobs, long commutes, and screen time. Prolonged sitting reduces muscle activity, lowers metabolism, and increases the risk of weight gain and insulin resistance.

◇ Practical Tips:

▪ Incorporate physical activity into your daily routine by taking short walks during breaks, using a standing desk, or scheduling regular exercise sessions.

▪ Find activities you enjoy, such as dancing, gardening, or playing sports, to make staying active more enjoyable and sustainable. Unhealthy Diets:

2. Processed foods, sugary beverages, and fast food options are often convenient but lack essential nutrients and are high in empty calories, sugar, and unhealthy fats.

◇ Practical Tips:
   - Focus on whole, nutrient-dense foods like fruits, vegetables, whole grains, lean proteins, and healthy fats.
   - Plan and prepare meals ahead of time to avoid relying on convenience foods.

- Experiment with new recipes and flavors to make healthy eating more exciting.
- Be mindful of portion sizes and pay attention to hunger and fullness cues to prevent overeating.

3. Excess Weight and Obesity

Obesity is a significant risk factor for Type 2 diabetes, as excess body fat can lead to insulin resistance and metabolic dysfunction.

◇Practical Tips:
- Set realistic weight loss goals and aim for gradual, sustainable progress.

- Focus on making small changes to your eating habits and physical activity levels rather than drastic, unsustainable measures.

- Seek support from a healthcare professional, nutritionist, or support group to help you stay motivated and accountable.

》Practical Tips for Lifestyle Modification:

1. **Get Moving:** Incorporate regular physical activity into your daily routine. Aim for at least 150 minutes of moderate-intensity exercise per week, such as brisk walking, cycling, or swimming. Break up long periods of sitting with short movement breaks throughout the day.

2. **Eat a Balanced Diet:** Focus on whole, unprocessed foods such as fruits, vegetables, lean proteins, whole grains, and healthy fats. Limit your intake of sugary snacks, refined carbohydrates, and high-fat foods. Be mindful of portion sizes and practice mindful eating to enhance awareness of hunger and fullness cues.

3. **Manage Stress:** Find healthy outlets for stress relief, such as meditation, deep breathing exercises, yoga, or spending time in nature. Prioritize self-care activities that promote relaxation and emotional well-being.

4. **Prioritize Sleep:** Aim for 7-9 hours of quality sleep each night. Establish a consistent sleep schedule, create a relaxing bedtime routine, and limit exposure to screens and stimulating activities before bed.

Chronic stress and inadequate sleep can disrupt hormone regulation, increase cortisol levels, and negatively impact blood sugar control.

◇ Practical Tips:

▪ Practice stress-reduction techniques such as mindfulness meditation, deep breathing exercises, or yoga to promote relaxation and mental well-being.

▪ Establish a consistent sleep schedule by going to bed and waking up at the same time each day, even on weekends.

▪ Create a calming bedtime routine that includes activities like reading, taking a warm bath, or listening to soothing music to signal to your body that it's time to wind down.

5. **Monitor Your Health:** Stay proactive about your health by scheduling regular check-ups with your healthcare provider. Monitor your blood sugar levels, blood pressure, cholesterol levels, and weight to track changes and identify potential risk factors early on.

By implementing these practical tips and making gradual, sustainable changes to your lifestyle, you can reduce your risk of developing diabetes and improve your overall health and well-being. Remember that every positive step you take towards a healthier lifestyle counts, and small changes can lead to significant long-term benefits.

Chapter 5

Navigating the Maze of Diet and Nutrition

When it comes to managing diabetes, what you eat matters—a lot. This chapter is your compass through the maze of diet and nutrition, where we debunk myths, outline practical strategies, and help you navigate toward a balanced and diabetes-friendly eating plan.

》Addressing Common Misconceptions about Diabetes and Nutrition

Misinformation about diabetes and nutrition is widespread, leading to confusion and frustration. Don't get caught up in the confusion. Let's clear the fog:

♤ **Sugar is the Enemy:** While it's true that sugary foods can cause rapid spikes in blood sugar levels, it's important to understand that carbohydrates are the main nutrient that affects blood sugar. Carbohydrates are broken down into glucose, which enters the bloodstream and raises blood sugar levels. This includes not only obvious sources of sugar like candy and desserts but also foods like bread, pasta, and rice.

♤ **You Must Avoid Carbs:** Carbohydrates are a crucial source of energy for the body, and they should not be completely eliminated from your diet. However, it's important to choose complex carbohydrates that are high in fiber and low in refined sugars. Examples include whole grains like quinoa, brown rice, and whole wheat bread, as well as fruits, vegetables, and legumes.

♤ **All Fats Are Bad:** Not all fats are created equal. While saturated and trans fats found in fried foods, processed snacks, and fatty cuts of meat can contribute to heart disease and insulin resistance, unsaturated fats found in nuts, seeds, avocados, and olive oil can actually have health benefits. These fats can help improve cholesterol levels, reduce inflammation, and stabilize blood sugar levels.

♤ **Artificial Sweeteners are Always Safe:** While artificial sweeteners like aspartame, saccharin, and sucralose are marketed as sugar alternatives for people with diabetes, research suggests that they may still have negative health effects. Some studies have linked artificial sweeteners to weight gain, insulin resistance, and changes in gut bacteria. While they can be used in moderation as part of a balanced diet, it's important to be mindful of their potential impact on health.

》Creating a Balanced and Diabetes-Friendly Diet

Now that we've debunked some myths, let's explore how to build a diet that works for you:

♡ **Focus on Variety:** Eating a diverse range of foods ensures that you get a wide array of nutrients essential for good health. Fruits and vegetables provide vitamins, minerals, and antioxidants, while lean proteins like chicken, fish, tofu, and legumes offer essential amino acids. Whole grains like oats, barley, and quinoa provide fiber and complex carbohydrates, while healthy fats from nuts, seeds, and olive oil support heart health.

♡ **Mind Your Portions:** Portion control is important for managing blood sugar levels and preventing overeating, which can lead to weight gain and insulin resistance. Using measuring cups, food scales, or visual cues like the size of your palm or fist can help you gauge appropriate portion sizes for different foods.

♡ **Plan Ahead:** Meal planning can help you make healthier food choices and avoid impulse eating. Consider planning your meals and snacks for the week ahead, taking into account your schedule and nutritional needs. Having healthy options readily available can make it easier to stick to your diabetes management plan.

♡ **Monitor Your Blood Sugar:** Keeping track of your blood sugar levels can help you understand how different foods and lifestyle factors affect your diabetes management. Keeping a food diary or using a mobile app to log your meals, blood sugar readings, and physical activity can provide valuable insights into your health and help you make informed choices.

♡ **Stay Hydrated:** Drinking plenty of water throughout the day is important for staying hydrated and supporting overall health. Water helps regulate body temperature, transport nutrients, and flush toxins from the body. It can also help prevent dehydration, which can worsen symptoms of diabetes and lead to complications like kidney disease and urinary tract infections. Limiting sugary beverages like soda, fruit juice, and energy drinks can help reduce your intake of empty calories and added sugars.

By adopting a balanced and diabetes-friendly diet, you can take control of your health and improve your overall well-being. Remember, small changes can lead to big results over time. With dedication and perseverance, you can navigate the maze of diet and nutrition with confidence and clarity.

In the next chapter, we'll explore the importance of regular physical activity in managing diabetes and maintaining a healthy lifestyle. Get ready to move and groove your way to better health!

Chapter 6

Exercise

In Chapter 6, we'll explore the power of physical activity in managing and preventing diabetes. Exercise isn't just about losing weight or building muscles—it's a crucial tool in your arsenal for better health and diabetes management. Let's dive in!

The Role of Regular Physical Activity:

1. **Improves Insulin Sensitivity:** When you engage in physical activity, your muscles require more glucose for energy. To meet this demand, your body becomes more sensitive to insulin, allowing it to more effectively transport glucose from your bloodstream into your cells. This process helps to lower blood sugar levels and reduce insulin

resistance, a hallmark of type 2
diabetes.

2. **Helps Manage Weight:** Physical activity
is an essential component of weight
management. By burning calories
through exercise, you can create a
calorie deficit, which can lead to weight
loss or weight maintenance. Even small
reductions in body weight can have
significant benefits for individuals with
diabetes, improving blood sugar control
and reducing the risk of complications.

3. **Lowers Blood Pressure and
Cholesterol:** Regular exercise has
been shown to lower blood pressure
and improve cholesterol levels, both of
which are important factors in reducing
the risk of cardiovascular disease, a
common complication of diabetes.
Exercise helps to strengthen the heart
muscle, improve circulation, and
promote the dilation of blood vessels,
leading to better overall cardiovascular
health.

4. **Boosts Mood and Energy**: Exercise
has profound effects on mental health

and well-being. Physical activity stimulates the release of endorphins, neurotransmitters in the brain that promote feelings of happiness and euphoria. Regular exercise can help reduce symptoms of stress, anxiety, and depression, which are often more prevalent in individuals with diabetes. Additionally, exercise increases energy levels and enhances overall vitality, making it easier to cope with the demands of daily life.

Simple and Achievable Exercise Routines

1. **Walking:** Walking is a low-impact exercise that can be easily incorporated into your daily routine. Start by taking short walks around your neighborhood or during breaks at work. Gradually increase your pace and distance as your fitness improves. Aim for a brisk pace that elevates your heart rate but still allows for comfortable conversation.

2. **Strength Training:** Strength training exercises help build muscle mass,

improve bone density, and increase
metabolism. You can perform
bodyweight exercises such as squats,
lunges, push-ups, and planks, or use
resistance bands or free weights for
added resistance. Start with light
weights and gradually increase the
resistance as you become stronger. Aim
for 2-3 sessions per week, targeting all
major muscle groups.

3. **Swimming or Water Aerobics:**
   Water-based exercises are gentle on the
   joints and provide a full-body workout.
   Swimming laps or participating in water
   aerobics classes can improve
   cardiovascular fitness, strength, and
   flexibility. The buoyancy of water
   reduces the impact on your joints,
   making it ideal for individuals with
   arthritis or mobility issues.

4. **Yoga or Tai Chi:** Mind-body practices
   like yoga and Tai Chi focus on controlled
   movements, breathing techniques, and
   meditation. These practices can improve
   flexibility, balance, and relaxation, which
   are important for overall health and
   well-being. Start with beginner classes

or instructional videos and progress at your own pace.

5. **Dancing:** Dancing is a fun and enjoyable way to incorporate physical activity into your life. Whether you join a dance class, follow along with online tutorials, or simply dance around your living room, dancing provides cardiovascular benefits, improves coordination, and boosts mood. Choose music and dance styles that you enjoy, and don't be afraid to let loose and have fun!

Incorporating a variety of physical activities into your routine can help keep your workouts interesting and prevent boredom. Experiment with different types of exercise until you find activities that you enjoy and look forward to. Remember to listen to your body, stay hydrated, and modify exercises as needed to accommodate any physical limitations or health concerns. With consistency and determination, you can reap the countless benefits of regular physical activity and take proactive steps toward better diabetes management and overall health.

Chapter 7

Breaking Free from Medication Dependency

Now, we delve into the intricate relationship between medication management and lifestyle changes in the journey towards freedom from medication dependency. Let's explore the importance of medication adherence while embracing alternative therapies and lifestyle modifications.

Understanding the Importance of Medication Adherence

- Blood Sugar Control

  Medications prescribed for diabetes, such as insulin or oral medications like metformin, work to lower blood sugar levels and maintain them within a healthy range. Consistent adherence to medication regimens is crucial for achieving stable blood sugar control and reducing the risk of hyperglycemia (high blood sugar) and hypoglycemia (low blood sugar), both of which can have serious health consequences.

- Preventing Complications

Diabetes is associated with a range of long-term complications, including cardiovascular disease, kidney disease, neuropathy (nerve damage), retinopathy (vision problems), and foot complications. Adhering to prescribed medications can help prevent or delay the onset of these complications by maintaining optimal blood sugar levels and minimizing fluctuations that can damage blood vessels and organs over time.

- Maintaining Quality of Life

Effective medication management can enhance quality of life for individuals with diabetes by minimizing symptoms such as excessive thirst, frequent urination, fatigue, and blurred vision. By stabilizing blood sugar levels, medications can help individuals feel better physically and emotionally, allowing them to engage more fully in daily activities and pursue their goals and interests.

- Stabilizing Mood and Energy

  Some diabetes medications, particularly those that regulate insulin levels or enhance insulin sensitivity, can have secondary effects on mood and energy levels. By improving blood sugar control and stabilizing hormonal fluctuations, medications can help individuals experience more consistent energy levels, mood stability, and overall well-being.

What Alternative Therapies and Lifestyle Changes Can Really Improve This Condition?

1. **Diet and Nutrition:** Adopting a balanced diet that emphasizes whole, nutrient-dense foods can have a profound impact on blood sugar control and overall health. Focus on consuming plenty of fruits, vegetables, whole grains, lean proteins, and healthy fats

while limiting refined carbohydrates, added sugars, and processed foods. Pay attention to portion sizes, meal timing, and carbohydrate intake to optimize blood sugar management.

2. **Physical Activity:** Regular exercise is essential for improving insulin sensitivity, enhancing glucose uptake by muscles, and promoting overall cardiovascular health. Aim for at least 150 minutes of moderate-intensity aerobic activity or 75 minutes of vigorous-intensity aerobic activity each week, in addition to muscle-strengthening activities on two or more days per week. Choose activities that you enjoy and that fit your fitness level and physical abilities.

3. **Stress Management:** Chronic stress can contribute to elevated blood sugar levels, insulin resistance, and inflammation, all of which can worsen diabetes symptoms and increase the risk of complications. Explore stress-reduction techniques such as mindfulness meditation, deep breathing exercises, progressive muscle relaxation, and guided imagery to

promote relaxation, reduce stress hormone levels, and improve overall resilience to stress.

4. **Sleep Hygiene:** Adequate sleep is essential for regulating hormone levels, supporting metabolic health, and promoting overall well-being. Aim for 7-9 hours of quality sleep per night and prioritize good sleep hygiene practices, such as maintaining a consistent sleep schedule, creating a relaxing bedtime routine, and optimizing your sleep environment for restorative rest.

5. **Support Networks:** Building a strong support network can provide invaluable emotional, practical, and informational support for managing diabetes and navigating the challenges of medication management and lifestyle changes. Seek out friends, family members, healthcare professionals, and diabetes support groups who can offer encouragement, understanding, and guidance on your diabetes journey.

By integrating medication adherence with lifestyle modifications and alternative therapies, you can optimize your overall health and well-being, reduce the risk of complications, and achieve greater control over your condition. Working collaboratively with healthcare providers and adopting a holistic approach to diabetes management can empower you to lead a fulfilling and active life while effectively managing diabetes.

Chapter 8

Say No to Diabetes - A Holistic Approach

In this final chapter, I summarize the essence of our journey through this book and advocate for a holistic approach to diabetes management. I'll reiterate the key takeaways from our exploration while I strongly encourage you to embrace a comprehensive approach to living well with diabetes.

Summarizing Key Takeaways from the Book:

1. Knowledge is Power: Understanding diabetes—its causes, symptoms, complications, and treatment options—is the first step toward effective management. By empowering yourself with knowledge, you gain the tools and confidence to take control of your health.

2. Lifestyle Matters: Diet, exercise, stress management, sleep hygiene, and other lifestyle factors play pivotal roles in diabetes management. Making healthy choices and adopting positive habits can significantly impact blood sugar control, overall well-being, and quality of life.

3. Medication Management: While lifestyle changes are important, medications also play a crucial role in diabetes management for many individuals. Adhering to prescribed medications and working closely with healthcare providers to optimize treatment regimens are essential components of effective diabetes care.

4. Mind-Body Connection: Recognizing the interconnectedness of physical health, mental well-being, and emotional resilience is key to holistic diabetes management. Strategies such as mindfulness, stress reduction, and cultivating a positive mindset can enhance overall health outcomes.

5. Support Systems: Building a strong support network of healthcare professionals, family members, friends, and peers can provide invaluable encouragement, guidance, and accountability throughout the diabetes journey. Seeking support and sharing experiences can foster a sense of community and empowerment.

A Holistic Approach to Diabetes Management:

Now, as we conclude our journey together, I encourage you to embrace a holistic approach to diabetes management—a philosophy grounded in the integration of knowledge, lifestyle changes, and ongoing support. Here's how you can embark on this transformative path:

1. Educate Yourself: Continue to seek knowledge and stay informed about the latest advancements in diabetes care, treatment options, and self-management strategies. Empower yourself with information and be proactive in advocating for your health.

2. Embrace Lifestyle Changes: Embrace the power of healthy habits and lifestyle modifications. Make nutritious food choices, engage in regular physical activity, prioritize stress management and self-care, and prioritize quality sleep. Small changes can yield significant improvements in your health and well-being.

3. Partner with Your Healthcare Team: Cultivate a collaborative relationship with your healthcare providers, including doctors, nurses, dietitians, and diabetes educators. Work together to develop personalized treatment plans, set realistic goals, and track progress over time.

4. Seek Support: Reach out to support groups, online communities, and peer networks for encouragement, guidance, and solidarity. Share your experiences, learn from others, and celebrate victories together. Remember, you are not alone on this journey.

5. Celebrate Progress: Celebrate your achievements, no matter how small. Recognize the effort and dedication you invest in managing your diabetes and prioritize self-compassion and self-kindness along the way.

By embracing a holistic approach to diabetes management—one that integrates knowledge, lifestyle changes, and ongoing support—you can reclaim control over your health and well-being. Say no to diabetes by saying yes to a life filled with vitality, resilience, and hope.

As you embark on this new chapter of your diabetes journey, remember that each step you take brings you closer to a brighter, healthier future. Together, let's continue to say no to diabetes and yes to living life to the fullest.

Thank you for joining me on this empowering journey. Wishing you strength, resilience, and abundant health on the road ahead.